MW01258602

I've Got Cancer, But It Doesn't Have Me!

A Survivor's Book of Poems

Copyright ©1995 by Barbara Whipple

◯ Full Moon Press ∼ Illinois

Post Office Box 91
Westmont, Illinois
60559
U.S.A.

A portion of the proceeds from this book will be donated toward cancer research.

All rights reserved. Except for appropriate use in critical reviews or works of scholorship, the reproduction or use of this work in any form or by any electronic, mechanical, or other means now known or hereafter invented, including photocopying and recording, and in any information storage and retrieval system is forbidded without written permission of the author.

ISBN 0-9647897-0-1

Library of Congress Catalog Card Number: 95-61869

Printed in the U.S.A.

10 9 8 7 6 5 4 3 2 1

I've Got Cancer, But It Doesn't Have Me!

A Survivor's Book of Poems

1/21/97

D.D.;
Thanks for being
my friend !
Barbara Whipple

By Barbara Whipple

Introduction

I was diagnosed with Stage III breast cancer in April of 1992. At the time, I was thirty-eight, married, and the mother of a four year old girl. After a modified radical mastectomy uncovered an eight centimeter tumor (the size of a baseball) and five positive lymph nodes, I've had four aggressive cycles of chemotherapy, an autologous bone marrow transplant, and a few other related minor surgeries. I'm still here. I'm in remission. I survived it. Hard to believe, as I look back.

But what's harder yet, is that all of what I went through is still sinking in. Statistically, I now have greater than a 50% chance of long-term survival, much better than the initial 18% chance I was given at the time of diagnosis. There is a high degree of probability that I have been cured by the bone marrow transplant—and that is my hope.

I have dreams of someday going back to live a simple life in a cabin in the woods, of writing more books and finishing my novel, and most importantly, of seeing my daughter grow up and sharing all those precious moments of her life with her. Sometimes I get overwhelmed by what has happened to me, and it's hard to plan for the future. Sometimes I feel like I'm living life on the edge. Sometimes, it's hard to think at all. But as my daughter now quips about everything, "You have to look on the bright side, mommy."

Today, I'm a licensed clinical social worker, with a bachelor's degree in psychology and a master's degree in social work. I've been a social worker since 1977, though I've always been involved with some kind of social service or social cause since the late '60s. I've always believed in the positive in people—I've always believed that together we could make the world a better place.

At this time in my life, I keep myself busy working full time as a high school social worker, mother, friend, writer, performance poet, and helping other cancer patients. I do whatever I can to keep myself occupied, including trying to find out what caused my cancer. I'm exhausted at times, yet energized. But I will not feel sorry for myself, and I'll do whatever it takes to escape that feeling.

The last six years haven't been easy: my mother died from leukemia; and both my former mother and father-in-law have died from liver cancer and lymphoma. My former brother-in-law is in remission from bladder cancer. My father tells me he has some form of skin cancer, but says not to worry. I look at my daughter, and pray that she will be spared this curse.

I recently discovered that I had once worked in a junior high school where 25 of the approximately 50 staff members have been diagnosed with cancer since 1978; and since 1991, of the thirteen cancers that were diagnosed, ten were breast cancer—including mine. But oddly enough, no one can explain why.

I've read that half of us will die from cancer. And then I get angry. Why isn't there a cure? What causes cancer?

But you'll have to do your own research, as I have. Read *Silent Spring* by Rachel Carson. Read everything you can. And then you'll find that there is only one choice—and that's to get involved. Because if it can happen to me, it can happen to you—and to the people you love.

And with that, welcome to the club—the same club to which Gilda Radner said she wished she didn't belong. But just because she didn't live, doesn't mean you won't. After all, look at me. Miracles happen.

Dedication

This book is dedicated to you, because whether you have cancer or not, you know someone who's had it. And fighting cancer is one of life's toughest battles, for everyone affected by it. Since my illness, many strong and courageous people have lost the battle—and many, many more still are here with us, living life to the fullest, taking each moment as it comes. What I have written here comes both from many dark nights, and from the bright sunlight showered on me by others. Whatever happens, you're not alone—just remember that.

I owe my life to Dr. Donald Sweet and everyone at Hinsdale Hematology/Oncology, for your caring and support, especially to Jan Wilson. To the staff at Hinsdale Hospital on 5 North, especially Linda Wojotowicz, Joannie Engel and Maribeth Maney, thanks for hanging in there with me. You're the best.

This book is also dedicated to all my friends at Lyons Township High School who have so graciously helped me survive with their love, prayers, cards, food, blood, and platelets.

Special love to my dad, Bill, and my step-mother Jerry, my precious daughter Laura, step-sisters Diana Rollins and Donna Trimble, step-brother Jimbo Dukes, and to cousins Kim and Candy. And most of all to my beloved mother, who I dearly miss.

My warmest thanks to Beverley Furman, Nancy Ging, Anne Hyman, Lou Jacobs, Nancy Bly, Mark Slakter, Phil Brown, Betty Federer, Jan Boerman, Betty Jones, Delores Lindgren, Romelle Marshall, Cathy Cahill, Sandy Coleman, Mary Baker, Lisa Starnes, Veronica Jean, Paul Greenberg, Byron Lee, Geralyn Ignarski, Jerry Martin, the Oswald family, Barb & John Maxwell, Ora Hoshen, Jeanette Belletire, Fred Jacobs, Ray Ku, Cliff Brickman, Irwin & Becky Myers, Duke

& Mimi Anderson, Kevin DuBrow, Jim & Roberta Ritter, Nancy Lennon, Nancy Evans, Anne Palmer, Kathy Nicoll, Francesca Valiani, Dorothy Kavka, the Union Church of Hinsdale, Clarendon Hills Care In Action, John Mahoney, Joe & Jeanne Nowak, Char Poelsterl, Joyce Tumea, and the Downers Grove Writer's Workshop.

This book is also very much dedicated to Stevie Nicks—my inspiration.

Contents

The Pearl

The doctor came in with the news
lips moving in slow motion
eyes unblinking
voice sober and flat
his world a gray clinical landscape;
mine, an inward journey
deep into the existential void
a communion with the cold kiss of death
where no one can ever return the same

his vacant stare watched through sterile curtains
of measured words
and noncommittal phrases;
unaskable questions
were answered with surgical succinctness,
but only a single word
that I understood
dropped from his thin lips over and over again...

he stood there, a priest
stuffed in an antiseptic white jacket
unable to offer redemption
from the large swollen lump and the stainless-steel
statistics that took each breath away...
I wondered if I were alive, if this were all real
as the moments ticked louder in my head
the spectre of death sucking in and out of my lungs
horror beyond horror consuming me
one centimeter at a time.

the masked fortune tellers in surgical gowns
rushed me down the hallway
into the morphine dream,
until I awoke

the milk-white pearl of my breast
ripped from its shell
the hot alien pain of amputation,
the alpha and omega
of what once was and will never be again
of what is to come.

I told them—slash me,
burn me,
poison me,
baptize me...purify me—my body is yours
I'll do anything you want
I just don't want the beast to chase me
through the shadows anymore
I only want to feel the cool earth
between my toes again
to dance naked in the woods
and see my child become a woman—
to feel hope once again.

Sandcastle

Depression hangs around my neck
a noose tightening
a ghoul stalking me
it haunts me through all the days
and the sleepless nights that seem to go on forever
I have built more than just a wall
I have built a fortress of denial
hardened like a brick inside
the laughter has become glue in my throat
the tears a fist in my heart
I cannot let go
cannot cry
or I will crumble
and fall
as fragile as crystal
and my strength will turn to sand
but I need to be in this place right now
for my pain binds me together
fortifies me
and keeps me focused on what I need to do
to be a victor
not a victim.

Stuck

How far down can you go
before you come up again?

How much can you suffer
until it's too much?

Cancer is the nightmare of nightmares—
it takes your life away
and never gives it back;

it is so powerful
your mind collapses in on itself
until you can't think
            can't remember
                        can't plan
so soundless it moves in like a fog
and whispers uncertainty
with its subtle sadistic evil
until it becomes panic
ringing
in your ears
                        yet

it is only when you reach a crisis
and drop to the lowest point
that shakes you to your roots
and leaves you
quivering against the wind
that you are compelled to look at yourself
re-evaluate your life
and the comfort of your complacency—
it forces you to move
            to act
                        to change
            to take the great leap of faith
                        and fly.

Yin/Yang

Black is the sum total
of all colors
combining
each blocking the other out
obscuring the purity
creating a reality of its own
essence
the absurd avant garde dance
music without composition
noise without vision
maturity is neither fighting nor running away
but making peace
learning tolerance
accepting the blend and the separation
the darkness and light
comprehending the structure of anarchy
in the universe
and the yin/yang shapes on the face
of the full moon
at night.

Insomnia

In the ice hot hiss of night
I cannot sleep in the twilight of twisted sheets
and dreamless thoughts
I can only stay awake and think
of some way to move forward
of some way to unlock this paralysis
to fulfill my dreams
get what I want
and do what I came here to do.

The Well

Curious,
I stare way over into
the big black bottomless pit
of the future
my fingers strain to pull me closer
and lean me over
further down
down into it
that wide cavernous mouth
it gapes wide open at me
smiling, inviting
eager to consume me
to melt my flesh into bone
into ash
into dust
and become earth again...

I bend further over as it pulls me in
to see more than I can look at
and know more than I want to know;
the well hypnotizes me like a crystal ball
luring me to leap
to fly away into another space less painful
less black and bottomless
to embrace the stars
and feel the sun steam through me
bursting with life into death
not tumbling down a long black well
deep into the oblivion of darkness.

But there is no bottom deeper
than this dark hole
sucking out all the light;

and there is no cry more mad than the screech
that tears from my lungs,
each breath emptier than the last...
Yet there has to be some meaning to this,
I must believe
I can feel it
I'm certain
as I open myself up
to the holy healing light
the brightness streaming down
penetrating the blackness
rescued at last
from the dark stranger in the mirror
illuminating this face
as distant and as familiar as the moon.

Where Are You?

This really isn't so bad
consider the alternative
isn't it wonderful
what technology can do nowadays
God?
where are you?

are you in the frozen bags of harvested marrow
in the anti-biotics and growth factor drugs
in the injections,
the computerized chemo machines,
or in the two catheters sewn in my chest?

are you here
in this tiny sterile room
with me
while I throw up and all my hair falls out
or do you float in and out
through the sleeping pills and tranquilizers
in the daydreams that pass
like ghosts in the night
or are you hiding
in the nightmares that awaken me
with every sunrise?

are you in the mist of the chaplain's eyes
looking at me with that piteous stare,
or are you in
the blood and platelets that keep me alive
in the drugs,
in my soul,
in the future...
is there something they're not telling me?
am I going to die

God?
will I go through all this in vain?

are you there?

and then I look out the fifth floor window
through the sweeping oaks that overlook
the park
their leaves blushing and curling with the fall
drifting in spirals to the earth
blowing and scattering across the grass
seeds of the future
yet unborn life awaiting spring
and I feel the wind fill me
stirring me
and in the quiet center of my mind
I feel you
and the inner wisdom
that I will survive.

To a Friend

How can I write
and explain all the pain?
Is it fair to tell you that my mind, my heart,
my soul is starving
and the world has nothing left to offer except raw bone.
I am a fragment of who I once was
ravaged by this disease
faint with fear
as I cling to the moment
and emptiness claws at me from inside.
I cannot capture the beauty anymore
for all the light and the joy has disappeared
and I am blinded;
but now more than ever
I need to see and find my way —
not feel lost in this desolate place
still searching people's faces for my salvation.
I know I must turn and face myself instead
and look forward
no matter how horrible it is
I only ask one thing...
that no matter what happens
just please remember me
please remember that I've tried
I've fought
I've done everything I can —
I refuse to give up.

The Question

Where do you go
when you meet a dead end
do you return to the beginning
and try to find another way
or do you just sit and wait
for someone to find you
and build fires of hope?

I decided to build a ladder of dreams
so I could see all the different ways
I could get there
and know which direction
I wanted to go.

Simple Gifts

It is the things that can't be seen
that can't be bought
and priceless beyond measure
hope, love and time
health, happiness, and peace
there are no substitutes
no riches except that
which exists in the heart.

For Charlotte

I thought my world was destroyed
the day you died
in six weeks I watched the cancer reduce you
to a tin of ashes
a magnificent woman
a beauty
a queen
my hero
there are no words to define a relationship like ours
the love of a mother and child
it is eternal
larger than life
imprinted on the mind
etched in the heart
held in the soul.
You gave me life
immeasurable in meaning
and I beheld your radiance...
your grace, your dignity
your courage
how can I thank you,
the purest rose of all roses
now but dried petals fallen
and crushed beneath the ground.

Dad

You're almost eighty now
the weathered wrinkles and spots of age
still outline the thousands of smiles
and millions of words we've shared
the jokes
the discussions
the truths
of who we are and what was important
are as imprinted in me
as they are on you
time has eroded
all dreams and disappointments
and we are both father and child
as we share
what time we have left with each other
before we part
and our hearts still long
for the woman who left us here
now alone together
the one who connected us
in the triad
the one who made you
my dad.

Hope

We can only live in the moment
we can only live in the now
yesterday has slipped away
and evaporated
no clearer or alive than a dream
vanished into thin air with a primeval poof
the magic of time
is the space that separates pain into segments
and allows us to forget
we start over again every day
every sunrise is new
and yet the sun remains the same
vibrant warm orange ball
that gives us energy
gives us life
the light pours into us
igniting the vision
and our ability to see
but if we look too far ahead
we can't enjoy where we are now
and if we look backwards
we cannot see where we're going
the mortality of every second
is the kindest gift of all —
the hope
that reaches
beyond the unbearable.

Relapse

It isn't the cancer that eats away at me
anymore
it isn't the memories
or the scars
that remind me of what I've been through
it is the fear
the anxiety feeding on every shallow breath
and the tickertape of doom running through my mind
I can't stop thinking about it
I can't believe I have cancer
this wasn't supposed to happen to me
there must be some kind of mistake
this happens to other people
people I don't know
you know, the ones in the National Enquirer
certainly not to real people,
not to me.
The shivering arches way up my spine
like a giant rollercoaster ready to drop
I don't know how I'm going to make it
through this
I don't know if I can take any more
but all I can do now is grit my teeth and hang on
and chant my silent mantra
and scream my silent scream
but the only way I can make this horrible feeling stop
is to do something for someone else
think of someone else
something positive
randoms acts of kindness
that I can give as gifts
and when I stay in the now
I don't have to think about the future
or feel the fear.

zen

The restlessness tingles
into my fingertips
like the deep gong of a bell
it quivers down my spine
and touches the souls of my feet
and sparks from my toes.
The world is shifting
and I must constantly adjust my stance
always moving
even when I want to be still
for I must remain strong
and not give up
standing upright.

How can I believe in a god
who has taken so much
and brought nothing but pain —
is there beauty in the agony of crucifixion
in the vacuous silence
that speaks my name?
Where are the answers
the promises not kept —
I would rather die as I stand
than sell out for some false security,
that insidious trickster who makes us
whores for our fear.

I still believe.

Jan-ism

It had to come out
I couldn't keep it in any more
for cancer is more than a disease
of the body
it eats away at your soul
if you let it
so I just sat there and sobbed
about every horrible thing
that had happened in my life
and how scared I was that I would die
just like my mother
but Jan said only five words
in her soothing voice
firm with conviction
"cancer is a do-able thing"
she smiled as she held my hand
and for the first time
I realized
I was going to live
after all.

Jerry

She comes to my hospital room every day
with a broad smile
and a sealed plastic bag full of pennies
bleached in Clorox for two hours
thoroughly washed and rinsed
sanatized and germ-free
and a crisp new deck of red Bicycle cards
she pulls from her purse
and remembers what day it is when I ask
what time it is
and tries to guess
whose turn it is to play
the next card
in the long sleepy afternoon
playing Kings on the Corner
enjoying the time and
the ritual of normalcy
joking about the food
and whatever else
I can't remember with my chemo brain
nor do I want to
but she just smiles
and we laugh just like children
playing a simple game
we don't keep score
we can't remember
we just keep throwing the pennies in
...yet I always seem to win.

The Plague

There are some poems that
cannot be written
some words that just cannot be said
pain is relative
painlessness is a form of bliss
for in this world
we were born to suffer
and to die
and to not suffer
is to know heaven...
I am not ashamed to tell you
that I am depressed
yet angry enough to fight the same grisly shadow
hollowed in my mothers fading eyes
in the blueness of her fingertips
and the blackness of her tongue
as she took her last breath...
and stopped...
the glow of her release still haunts me
but I couldn't hold her until she was gone
and the warmth drained from her skin
couldn't tell her how much it hurt
how much she had meant to me
until now —
and I thank God
she never knew what has happened to me.

Survival

I run here
and there
as though I had somewhere
important to go
but the reality is
there is no important place to go
or things to do
there is only now
the moment
this moment
and that I'm alive —
nothing else matters.

Who I Was

I look over the past and
try to determine
what was so all important
back then
to identify the facts
the events
the turning points
the feelings that formed me
into who I am
my character
my substance
but tomorrow will come
as it always does
and I don't know
who I'll be
then
but it won't matter
anyhow
for a hundred years from now
no one will ever know I lived
no one will care
about someone they never knew
the only people who really matter
are the people I love
and me
now
for it is only the love
that survives.

Winter

It is winter
the cold swoops down
a vulture clawing into me
piercing to the bone
there is blood spilled here
on this white snow
and I am no longer a virginal little girl
I close my eyes to the white and the red
and search black
the tunnel leading down the path
of long nights
and only the sound
a breath in and out
the blood swooshes
pulsing with my heart
the sweat pours off me
an explosion in my head
a supernova of stars crackling
before my very eyes
I am faint
I cannot speak
I can only sink
down
into the cold and snow
buried in darkness
the coccoon of silence surrounding me
immobilized by my weakness
until I grow
and mature enough
to push back the cold
stand up and leave
to only go
where it's warm.

God

I woke up early this morning
hanging on to the faint edge of a dream
grasping at the final fading images
slipping into consciousness
from the ripening hum of absolute solitude
the faces emerged
from all the long forgotten memories
taking form
connecting parts of myself that had been missing
parts I could never explain
converging into the same stream
with the buddha consciousness
of reincarnation
not of body
but of that which we can only know
in the collective energy of the spirit
for the serenity of the wilderness
is as vast as the passionate color of a flower
that touches us
and once we know
we can never forget
not even in the final dreamless
painless sleep of death
where God waits
to bring us home.

The Transplant

Death comes as a doorknock
black veils and the sweet sick smell of flowers
a skeleton with a smile
offers an invitation to the infinite dark dance
the groom of eternity seeks to walk me down the aisle
toward the altar of the absurd
the music in the background is but a question
can this really be happening to me?
the final thoughts
the final gasp of comprehension
that I am letting go of everything
I have ever known or loved
my fate sealed
with the cosmic kiss of chemo
my destiny
has finally made meaning
out of the meaningless
and found God in a godless world
I close my eyes and do not listen
to the scary rapping deep in my wooden heart
I take a long deep breath and sigh
seeking my center
knowing that I must be strong
and that I will soon dance.

Why Me?

I used to think
what's wrong with me
why do I always do things
the hard way
and everything bad
always seems to happen to me.
I had chosen not to write
the story of my life
part of me still
had a need to be perfect
and avoid the other parts
the broken parts
the imperfect parts
and to start is to finish
to complete is to admit
mortality...
but as I stare up at the Milky Way
swirling above me
I know we are all immortal
in our own mind's eye
and I have become the Buddha woman
who reflects upon the lake
the waves lap upon the shore
like the tongues of a thousand thirsty wolves
reaching down from the belly of the moon.

Luck

Some people get lucky
and live life the easy way
they get what they want
and want what they get
their life is simple
happy
carefree
but
no matter what I do
it's hard
from crisis to crisis
nightmare to nightmare
the curse reappears in every form
lurks like a shadow
a vapor of extinction waiting for me
but
I am not one of the 35,000 children
sick and starving to death every day
in this world
I am lucky
for all that I am
and all that I have
and for the gift of time I have been allowed
to have lived this long
to have known what I know
and the unconditional love I have been given
is a blessing
a greater joy than just luck
a greater happiness
a greater sense of peace.

The Joy

Laura
how sweet you are
my precious little one
I love you more than I could love anyone
for you are all that is beautiful
to me
tender flower
dancing in the wilderness
floating across ice like an angel
cherub cheeks and rosebud lips
your wild brown hair is a mane
that trails behind you like a wedding veil
as you jump and spin
joyous virgin
unspoiled
innocent
loving
happy
child
for six and a half years
the tight hugs you have given me
are like bunches of flowers
I will always hold in my heart
everfresh, everspecial, everyou
you are the greatest gift of life
every day I love you more deeply
every precious moment more closely
knowing that nothing can separate us
for we are the same flesh
the same heart
the same spirit
no matter what happens

I will always be with you
will love you forever, my sweet daughter,
my little girl.

Coping

I am weary of talking
today I wish just to stay home and putter
around the garden
and only do things for me
I am happy
knowing I am not alone
anymore than anyone else
this comedy of terror
has confined me too much
and not let myself be vulnerable
to risk or fear
I want to touch each tender petal of the flower
and inhale the nectar from its being
to dig my fingers deep into the earth
and turn the soil
plant new life
and watch it grow.

Resolution

In the quiet of night
I escape from the darkness
and stare up at the stars scattered across the sky
like glitter
for a single flickering moment
the image connects me to you
and we are but a flash of humanity
breathing and sighing as the world labors
silently onward
where nothing stands still
and nothing stays the same.
No matter where you are
that is where you are meant to be;
all we can do for each other is to hold hands
and hold on tight.
My sadness once was so deep
that if I could cry
I'd never have stopped—
and all I had gone through
would have been in vain.
There's only once choice
to live
or die.
I have cancer
but it doesn't have me.

Snow

The snow comes down
each flake drifting
on its own current
its own path
its own pattern
it falls from heaven
a single droplet of water
transformed
into a jewel
that whirls and dances through space
and time
until it becomes
water once again.

Recovery

I don't think I'll ever recover what I lost
but I don't think I would have ever gained so much
without giving up what I had

I spent twenty-six days in isolation
in the bone marrow unit
thinking about what I would do
with the rest of my life if I should survive

I have always had goals in my life
always had something I would look forward to
always had remorse about opportunities lost

I spent every day up there
seeing the world through sterile masks and rubber
gloves
my body dying from the inside out
and from the outside in
but somehow all of those goals and opportunities
didn't matter anymore

so I made plans
just to make it through the day.

Physical Therapy (For Romelle)

You've worked me over
challenged my limits
and my threshold of pain
we've shared each other's trust
the confidences
and difficult moments in our lives
yet you still push and pull
tug and twist
put me on hot pads
then slap on the ice
yank and bend me
and knead out the knots
but if I resist
there's no mercy
and you press hard
to soften the scars.

Who I Am

Somehow I write
what's important
to make a statement
that no one can ever change
once it's printed
not even me
for the words
are written as with the strokes of a brush
intricate and refined
the image is art
with meaning
a life of definition and perspective
background highlighting foreground
shadows creating light
we view the world
in three dimensions
yet live the fourth in time
every moment an interpretation
an evolution of who we are.

Quality

I think back over my life
and remember what it was that meant something
that was outstanding
of quality
and had value
I muse at all the unexpected moments
of beauty
and tenderness
of surprises and twists and turns
that somehow worked out right
the risks that gave back more
than hoped for—my daughter
my family
those intense heartfelt talks late into the night
letters of encouragement and hugs from friends
love
fellowship
community
all the causes for peace and justice
fought so long and hard for
and won
I recall all the music and the concerts
the books and movies
every person who opened my mind
I remember one early morning in the pre-dawn forest
listening to the wilderness
an instant so pure
feeling the tears of elation
how can I feel that I've lost anything
how can I pity myself
having all the greatness that has been given to me

or regret every gift of breath
and moment of contentment;
I must be thankful —
and now,
I must be brave.

The Novel

I've been working on a book
since 1978
that emerged from a life-changing experience
of working in a therapeutic community
called Wolf Lake Refuge
deep in the northwoods of Minnesota
once translated into two inadequate screenplays
and numerous edited manuscripts
several times numbering over three hundred pages
a full-length novel
I have never been able to complete
and yet cannot ever stop writing;
I am compelled to tell this story
of a journey I took in my early twenties
as a social worker from inner-city Chicago
into the great wooded wilderness surrounding a pristine
lake
for nearly two years of my life
I worked and struggled
with a group of visionaries
carving out a common dream
building a community
of social service and education and reverence for the
earth —
part of me still has never returned
to this modern technosociety
even though the Refuge lies far away and abandoned
now
painfully given back to
and reclaimed by the forest
victim of budget cuts and political maneuvering
I must continue to write

and try to tell the story
of what we did
what we shared
what we believed
because the strength and intensity
of what I learned there
meant and gave me something more
than I have ever experienced
and I must keep the vision alive.

Dreams

I had dreams when I was young
that I thought would come true
I believed that if I wished hard enough
and did my best
I would get what I wanted
and if I were good
I would be happy for the rest of my life
and nothing bad would ever happen to me;
maybe I've never grown up
because I still have those dreams
when I look at my daughter peacefully sleeping
and try my best
to do everything right for her.

Detachment

Why is today better and the world feels lighter...
is it because I stepped back
and numbed myself to the negative;
or that I reframed and refocused
my approach,
my priorities,
and learned
to find the positive
I want to live
I want even much more than that
I refuse to let the cancer come back
and invade my life once more
I don't fear death...
I fear losing a life yet unlived, and
I don't want to live on the cliff anymore
with nowhere to turn
and no escape;
I must accept that
the hell we fear
is here in this place
on this planet
from the moment of birth
it follows us into the grave.
I must find comfort
in who I am and the life I have
in the priviledge of being here at all
to see beyond what is
to be thankful
and remember
to laugh.

One Second Till Midnight

I understand it all now
the evolution of this living planet
Gaia cell of cells
and we the cancer that feeds on it
the breast of earth is being sucked dry
cracking from the pressure
of too many mouths screaming to be fed
we anoint ourselves with organochlorines and DDT
and fill our bodies with preservatives and BHT
the nitrates of eternal life
we embalm the seas with styrofoam and plastic
and flatten the land as though it were our servant
we slaughter everything
with fuel emissions and plutonium —
biochemical warfare and cigarette smoke
suckle our need for power
our need to look cool —
money is the only green that's left
we've sold out everything
and we keep buying more
recycling the garbage
into designer drugs and cyberspace
we search for better, cheaper substitutes
for community
for soulmates and substance
for meaning
and the sense of belonging in a lost world
we are feeding ourselves false truths
and half realities
drunk with desire and denial
we are killing ourselves and our children

and soon there will be nothing left —
we must either change our attitude, or die.
Come join me
I choose to stand and fight—
we have nothing left to lose.

Prisoner

I am caught in a cage
I have built for myself
addicted to the narcotics
of the material world
yet a refugee
on a journey inward
I follow the trail of my spirit
searching dreams back to their origin
and I become the wolf woman once again
hungering for liberation
pacing back and forth on the path
going in circles
contemplating redemption
tearing off the garments of civilization
with a paw caught in a trap
grunting and groaning
wailing and howling
to merge and give birth
to know fullness
the final joy
before I can run free.

Nirvana

The absence of color is white
pure essence of simplicity
basic and true to its own nature
uncomplicated
unstructured
known only by the inner spirit
by gentleness
and quiet.

Snow White

I want to cast off
all the possessions
that tie me to machines;
the more I produce
the more I invest
the more I want,
bound in the cycle of addiction
compulsive slave to obsession
the need to have
the gluttony in us hungers
we are buyers and sellers,
dazzled by the shiny new young
sleek sophisticated
glamorous expensive beautiful
sexy
handsome muscular
modern hip hot cool and politically-correct
techno upgraded revised
award-winning expensive
prestigious designer
low-fat low-cal anorexic gourmet
of the milk-white homogenous material world
feasting on the repackaged poisoned apple,
we trade commodities
endlessly sleepwalking the yellow-pages of civilization
with nothing left to wake us
except the kiss of death
to see if there's anything worthy of saving
left inside.

You

How can I show you the moon
so you will always be able to see it
how can I give you joy
so you will always know it
how can I capture time
so that you can always have it
how can I share my life
so I will know that you can always remember it
I want to give you my love
so you will always feel it
and even though all points of our life have converged
into one perfect orb
etched into the transcendent universe
of this one brief moment in time
the fingers of skin on skin
and soul touching soul
I still want to climb into your eyes
and reach in as far as anyone could go
and make a home in your heart
and know we will be together forever
and there will be no more pain.

Social Responsibility

Hear the distant voices
wooden flutes and pulsing drums
echoes whispering on the wind
the scent of sweetgrass and juniper
lingers everywhere
sweatlodges and moondances
tell tales we cannot comprehend
the sense of community now decimated
the slaughter of the tribe
pulls at us like a dream
we can't forget
and all that remains
are the stumps
of trees
a forest

clear-cut.

The Dream

It seems that over the years
through the changes
beyond the doubts and heartache
a dream
the same dream
tugs at me like a conscience
always returning me to the center
of my existence
to a feeling of fullness
a connectedness of purpose and action
of meaning and triumph over adversity
that what I do is worthy
honorable
and just —
I think back to the heroes who have molded me
and through their character
have shown me the way
to a higher level of perceiving
a deeper level of feeling
compassion
social justice
and the strength to stand up
for what's right
even when there's no solid ground
even if I have to stand alone.

Jessica

I remember when I first met you
and how close to my age you were
sitting in the waiting room of Dr. Sweet's office
nervously flipping through the pages
of a faceless magazine
and I twiddling my thumbs
waiting
I tried not to notice the few remaining dull wisps of
hair under your hat
just like mine
your sallow grayish skin
eyebrowless eyes
or your hoarse gravelly voice
as you smiled and said hi when I first sat down...
I think I might have spoken first after that
and we talked for a long time about our lives
our cancers
our chances for survival
and our young children
there was so much we seemed to have in common
so much we shared
through our fear and our fight
like instant karma
the energy radiated between us in that short time
a warmth that bonded us to the future
to the hope that both of us could make it
and survive
I finally asked how things were going
and you so relieved to finally be in remission
but wishing to get rid of the pleurisy
that had settled in your chest and in your throat
we chatted on and on

finding in each other someone who really knew
what it was like to have cancer
and to be winning
but then you had to go in for your appointment
and I went in for mine,
and I only saw you twice after that
though it was really a lifetime
up in the bone marrow unit
trying to destroy the tumor that turned out not to be
pleurisy
but instead
the cancer
that destroyed you.
I miss you, Jessica.
I'm sorry.

Fantasy

I wake up in the morning and roll over
the sun and light wisps of spring wind
and chirping of birds
billow through the starchy white curtains
as I scrunch down in my cozy cotton bed
and yawn
I smell breakfast cooking downstairs
maple syrup and bacon everywhere
I hear the clatter of dishes and silverware
and the voices of my parents thrumming
while turning the pages of the newspaper
on another Saturday morning
when I am six.

Obituary

What will they say
what will they write
who would know
what really mattered
how do you summarize a life—
the colors are on the palette
but the picture is in the mind
a symbol of the spark
but not the spark itself
I don't care what people say about me
anymore
I don't care what they know
we all share the same secrets
hide the same fears
there is no pride or modesty
there is only you and me
and here and now
and what we choose
to do or waste.

Synchronicity

The first time I saw you
I knew
soul meeting soul
mind meeting mind
the harmonic convergence
was stronger than a magnet pulling us together
bonding us to a path we had to follow
seeking the treasure
we knew we had to find together
or be lost forever
alone
feeling that emptiness
never finding
peace.

1/20/97

I met with Mary Campbell this morning until 9:30 to discuss the Quest & Alternative program. I would like to schedule a follow-up meeting as soon as possible.

Barbara Whipple

Abundance

I never knew what hope really meant
it seemed to be something
that was used for somebody else
because it seemed so extreme
and hope was for the hopeless
like food was for the starving
and I had never starved before
until now
I have found that hope is vision
a gift that empowers
inspires
transcends
creates fullness —
the manna from heaven
becomes the fruit of the spirit.

The Refuge

I am swallowed by the wilderness
content just to stand and stare
my feet firm on the heavy damp forest floor
my eyes following wild iris petals
dripping purple everywhere
the sun rising a red flashing phoenix
from ashes of earth
to rainbow sky
the emerald groves of pine sit
tall silent buddhas
planted from seeds scattered by the wind
and the struggle of bird and beast
to survive
the patterns of language intertwine
they sing to me from their essence
with the dance of the stars
the land and trees kiss the heavens
and no barriers exist
between the moon and the planets
the howl of wolves and the cry of loons
and the wind
or I
will rise from the ashes of my life
and live
in the wildness
in the ancient community of nature
the tapestry of this kingdom
cradling my body in the breeze
rushing my hair about my face
feeling all that is in and around me.

Quantity

I'm tired most of the time
a real go-getter
penciling in the calendar
scheduling every moment
trying to figure out ways to fit everything in
trying to do it all
at the same time
doing double time
triple time
saving time
making the most of my time
but not taking the time,
my time.

Truths

Sometimes it comes out when I'm dressing
sometimes it comes out just anywhere
about the bad pill that made all my hair fall out
about the long times I spent in the hospital
about the breast that sometimes isn't there
she doesn't understand
why I am different
and I can't always do what other mommies do
but I tell her that everyone is different
and every time she looks at me I wonder
how to tell her
about this disease
and yet I hold back
the churning in my stomach
of not wanting
cancer to destroy her life, too
still so happy
so innocent
she is too young to understand
so instead I squeeze and kiss her
and tell her I love her
love her more than anything or anyone in the world
and that I will always be with her
no matter what happens
someday
I must tell her
that my life is tentative
or lie and tell her not to worry and that I am cured
keeping my fingers crossed
as we take our daily vitamins
warning her to be very careful
what she eats and breathes and touches

for someday soon she will have to know
the words I cannot speak right now
and she will have to be aware
and understand
it may as easily happen
to her.

The Dance

It isn't really about love
or obsession
the desire to have
to consume
to be a part of
need
want
or crave
it isn't seeking other people
other places
power
or money
it isn't related to beauty
fame
attractiveness
size
age
fitting in
or uniqueness
it has nothing to do with identity
politics
sexuality
success
individualism
strength of character
or wit
it doesn't matter where you've been
where you're going
or where you want to go
it has no relevance to what you know
who you know
or don't know

it has no color
no yesterday
no tomorrow
no beginning
and no end
it's just about your body
connecting with your spirit
and the music
playing endlessly in your head.

The Skater

I live for skating
yet I don't skate
every day I go to watch her
dance in her pretty pink and golden dress
I love to see her spin and twirl
the sparkles and colors flowing behind her
she jumps fearlessly
her smile leaping with her
as she winds her way around the rink
her blades glisten across the crisp white ice
cutting a new path
a new future
of combinations and possibilities
patterned after the lessons of the past
she loves to skate
so effortless
natural
graceful
ice ballerina
an angel given to me as a gift
and I've never felt such joy in what we share
knowing that she will never leave me
nor I leave her
for we were meant to be together
I, her guide and coach
she, my healer.

The Rose

I am trying to find
some way to offer you hope
some way to comfort the trembling
that shudders
through your bones
to the very center of your being
I want to tell you
that we can still dream of tomorrow
and hold hands
as though we'll never say goodbye
for all that we know and feel and desire
only exists in the moment
as does the fear
and pain
evaporates as quickly as it comes
for nothing can really harm us
except that which we allow inside our hearts
for all our time is limited
all our moments but a breath
a summer flower in bloom
we must enjoy the sunlight
to stretch toward the warmth
before we sink
back down into the moist darkness
withered by the winter of time
to await another season
another breath
the transition
the rebirth.

Alter Ego

How can I tell you what it means
to know you
for you have touched the full moon
I can see it in your eyes
the radiance like a jewel
hung forever in the velvet black sky
reflecting all the power within you
for to hear you sing
is to listen and know the soul
your magic pulls me up
and I am ready to leap through the lookinglass
and go to the other side
to fly away and embrace the light
to soar and feel the sun
burning through me until I am pure
smoke of the spirit
you are but a dream
a poet, a gypsy
an angel
travelling the universe on the wings of your voice
arcing as high as one can go
into the rapture of the cosmic dance
your crystal visions
are words that only the lonely could understand
and only pain could carve into the heart
I hear you
and know we have bled the same blood
sisters of the same moon
who have dreamt the same dreams
this life has brought us to our knees
and lifted our eyes toward heaven
I just wanted to thank you for helping me

you saved my life
and been there when I've been lost
you've given me hope
and kept me going
when I didn't feel like I could go on.

The Cure

Everyone's always looking for easy answers
to the hard questions
searching
willing to pay any price
for ways to numb the pain
if we could only make it go away
if only we could find some reasonable rationalizations
some artsy alternatives
cosmetic cures and designer drugs
far-out fantasies to believe in
to save us from the ache in our gut that won't disappear
we look away from the center
to the outside
to strangers and icons who promise relief
all the trendy charasmatic miracle workers
wolves in sheep's clothing
who take our money and feast on our anxiety
who testify their truth will heal
their skill will save
and connect us with higher powers
alien to our own experience
we must clear away all the foreign debris
that blocks our vision
take off the rose-colored glasses
and turn inward to face the clear hard truth
of who we are
and what we are
by accepting and forgiving
our own humanness
only then can we be real
to love ourselves and feel the love of others
to take risks and give who we are away —

that is the only force that can fill and heal us
and cure the loneliness and fear
of the death
we all must face someday.

Full Moon

A poem
as clear as a tear
a pearl
white shiny opalescent moon
jewel star hung in the sky
for all to see
and each to look within
for to know the soul
is to go as far as one can go
to go home
to find the mother within
the only comfort
the only joy
where there is nothing more to want
except to look forward
to the end of it all
to suffer no more
and cry no more tears —
I will be with you till the end
my friend
your golden face
and smiling glow
warms us all.

How To Live

Life isn't romantic
for those who must face it
it isn't glamorous
easy
or enchanting
and neither is death
but no matter what we do
we must experience both
how we became and
where we come from is as vague
as how we leave and where we will go
all of us are the blind
leading the blind
moving through the obscurity of space
where energy is neither created nor destroyed
we are to be transformed in the quantum leap
but we will never be the same
just as every day and moment differ while we live
change is the only reality we can count on
the only force we must reckon with
and God is the only power
who knows why.

My Doctor

Together
we search for comic relief
playing the limits of gallows humor
braving every topic
from the wonders of the growth factor drug
neupogen
a.k.a. Miracle Gro
to the potential of Chia Pet
for providing thicker coverage
on those more bald days

we've critically assessed
the latest styles and trends in
wigs
politics
breast reconstruction
cup sizes and cancer chic
as he patiently sits with me
listening closely
as though I were Jonas Salk or Einstein
I show him every article
ever written about cancer
carefully clipped from such pretigious publications
as the Journal of the American Medical Association
the New England Journal of Medicine
the National Enquirer
the Globe
and the Star

we debate the scope of possible causes
research on organochlorines
genetics
the meaning of cancer clusters

the intrinisc value of shark cartilage
decipher the reliability of statistics
and survival rates
explore the magnitude
of doing a national telethon
to find a cure
and he listens
listens as though he had no other appointments
and we were just friends
sipping lemonade
during a long willowy afternoon chat
out on the front porch

with a twinkle in his eye
his dry wit is a sponge that has soaked up
the multitude of my tears
he has held my hand
wiped my runny nose
looked at what no one wants to see
and saved my life
given me the priceless gift of
laughter
hope
the truth
and
there is no individual in all my life
I have ever known
to be as professional
caring
or kind
a true humanitarian
with a brilliant dash of spice.

Summary

I think back over all that happened
and know that it wasn't always that sad
that there is humor in anything
if you're willing to see it.
Before I went into the hospital
I only had a few sprigs of hair left
but my long-time hairdresser couldn't bring herself
to shave my head
so I went to the local barbershop instead
plopped down in the chair
lifted off my wig
and said
"just take it off the top"
which he did without a blink
as the eyes of the old men peered over
the tops of their newspapers
and tried not to stare.
And later when the other social workers
from work came by for a visit
I drove crazy Carl's phallic hot red Corvette
roaring around the streets
of the winding small town
without my wig on
as people gaped and took a second glance
at my shiny bald head and lipstick laughter flying by.
Sometimes I would say to people who
didn't know me well, "you want to see something?"
and then I'd lift my wig off
and for a moment they'd look around
to see if they were on Candid Camera.
And once I tossed my prosthesis to a friend
to hold so I could roll down a grassy hill

out in the country on a sublime summer's day.
Cancer has taught me to be spontaneous
to be more playful
more bold and daring
it has allowed me to live in the moment
and to do what I want
to be whoever I want to be
however I feel
a freedom that very few people have
and yet yearn for
a luxury I would never give up.

Encouragement

What is courage, you ask.
I say, face your fear,
the pain, horror—
get a grip
and hang on tight
believe you can make it
and do things for yourself
don't give up
go swim with the dolphins
it's too soon to run off into the woods and die
share all that you are and experience
know what being a family means
be a friend and be there for others
no matter how bad you feel
for you must live
and have faith in yourself
and in the universe...
you don't have to live with cancer
you can conquer it
that's why you're going through this
so believe that you're full, not empty
comfort your own trembling and stand firm
be a warrior,
a victor,
and be strong—
discover your power and use it
live in the here and now
reconcile with the past
and forget the future;
let go and say goodbye to what once was...
you have to move ahead
you have to live as all must live

without guarantees
so get tough
get going
waste no more precious time
and live it all.

ORDER FORM

A portion of the proceeds from this book will be donated toward cancer research.

Please send _____ copies of *I've Got Cancer, But It Doesn't Have Me! (A Survivor's Book of Poems)*

by Barbara Whipple, L.C.S.W. and cancer survivor.

$12.95 EACH Plus $3.50 shipping for the first book, and $1.00 for each additional book. Allow 4–6 weeks for delivery.

Number of books, times $12.95 _____
ILLINOIS RESIDENTS ADD $1.03 EA. (8.5% SALES TAX)

Plus Shipping $3.50 PLUS $1.00 PER ADD'L BOOK _____

TOTAL _____

TO ORDER CALL (800) 594-5190
OR SEND CHECK OR MONEY ORDER TO:

○ Full Moon Press ∼ Illinois
Post Office Box 91, Westmont, Illinois 60559 U.S.A.

NAME _____

ADDRESS _____

_____

CITY _____ **STATE** _____ **ZIP** _____

TELEPHONE (   ) _____

ORDER FORM

A portion of the proceeds from this book will be donated toward cancer research.

Please send _____ copies of *I've Got Cancer, But It Doesn't Have Me! (A Survivor's Book of Poems)*

by Barbara Whipple, L.C.S.W. and cancer survivor.

$12.95 EACH Plus $3.50 shipping for the first book, and $1.00 for each additional book. Allow 4–6 weeks for delivery.

Number of books, times $12.95 _____
ILLINOIS RESIDENTS ADD $1.03 EA. (8.5% SALES TAX)

Plus Shipping $3.50 PLUS $1.00 PER ADD'L BOOK _____

TOTAL _____

TO ORDER CALL (800) 594-5190
OR SEND CHECK OR MONEY ORDER TO:

◯ *Full Moon Press ∾ Illinois*

Post Office Box 91, Westmont, Illinois 60559 U.S.A.

NAME _____

ADDRESS _____

_____

CITY _____ **STATE** _____ **ZIP** _____

TELEPHONE (   ) _____

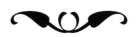